Healing through Happiness

Healing through Happiness

written and illustrated by
Donna Jane Sirlin

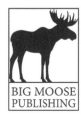

BIG MOOSE
PUBLISHING

Published by: Big Moose Publishing
PO Box 127 Site 601 RR#6 Saskatoon, SK CANADA S7K 3J9
www.bigmoosepublishing.com

ISBN: 978-1-989840-52-8 (hc)
ISBN: 978-1-989840-47-4 (sc)
Big Moose Publishing 07/23

What if healing
through happiness is
our birthright and the
purpose of life is to
have fun?

Prologue

"Wash your hands, sanitize everything, and ration your toilet paper."

Hello, global pandemic, a world of drama and trauma. It was March 2020, and the entire population was in lockdown.

It was a dreadful time, yet I found a way to be creative, and as a result of that choice, created something different. I found a way to heal myself through happiness. It became evident that time itself is nothing but change, and if you allow change to happen, everything can work out for you, possibly better than you can even imagine. What if there are no real problems, only possibilities? What if when challenged, we asked ourselves does it really have to be this way? What else is possible here?

How did the healing happen and why am I so happy?

It started with a generous share, a call to action by a friend on Facebook. She posted a video of a beautiful book she had created in her art class earlier in the year. In the video, she asked who would like to join her in a virtual art class.

ME! I chose that! It was a perfect setup.

I haven't taken an art class since I was 11 years old and I used to have a passion for art. I had forgotten how I loved working with my hands, working with color and texture. I loved acrylics and oils. I made beautiful woodwork and string art. I've seen pieces like the ones I used to make as a child, at recent art fairs and it would give me pause. So much had happened to that little girl who loved art and so much of her innocent joy was hidden away.

I soon received a box of supplies, which was like the best birthday present ever. I was so excited, it was overflowing with paint, ink, and unique art supplies.

Our first class began and for 5 weeks we worked on a different aspect of creativity and talked and expressed ourselves through Zoom and on our pages. It was the best medicine for the sickest of times. For me, it was like a cleansing of all the shock and trauma that was happening around me and the world.

When we completed, Patricia, the art teacher, asked if anyone wanted to go round 2 and that was a no-brainer. Again, I received the beautiful box of treasures and added a few of my own. Round 2 was where this book was born. It was raw and real and honest and authentic. I loved what it represented and how it made me feel. It's more than what meets the eye. I lovingly placed it on my cocktail table.

My book started to attract attention. Friends would sit and look through the pages, commenting so warmly and many in surprise and awe. I had always been told to write a book but write a book about what? People seemed to think I had something to share.

When a friend who had written a book said to me, "If I knew how you illustrated I would have had you do my book," it was an A-HA for me. She continued, "You should publish this." I asked her how would I start to transform this book of art into a "real" book.

That conversation set me on a journey of becoming an author and major self-discovery. At times it was an internal fight with myself, "What are you doing? This is silly; who do you think you are? You are wasting your time and your money".

You know those voices in your head.

The most transformative moments were when I said to myself, "Don't talk to me that way. I know who I am and I know what's right about this book". "I know that someone will pick it up and it will touch them as it has touched me to create it. I've seen the proof already so don't tell me to stop and that I can't do it. I'm doing it".

This was my healing through happiness.

So here we go.

What did you love to do as a child that you haven't done since then?

What brought you joy? What lights you up?

I would like to invite you, readers, to have a journal or a notepad and write what pops for you as you read this book. We all have hidden gifts and talents that we have buried or suppressed. I hope this starts to unhide yours and as we unhide together we can shine brightly our authentic light on the world.

Gratitude

I am very grateful to myself for being willing to choose greater, no matter what the conditions.

To Iris, through your generous sharing I was inspired to take this online art class.

To Patricia, the art teacher, you led me through this unknown process and created a space where I could reveal powers and potencies I didn't even know I had.

To those who admired, and were touched by, the art book project.

To Inessa, when you said, "If I knew you could illustrate I would have hired you to do my book." You really never know when a small action or a few words can change someone's life.

To Sara, the grand facilitator of consciousness, and empowerer of how to live your most unlimited life. I am so grateful for you and your Wings of Being program (www.wingsofbeing.com), which has inspired me to create even more magic in my life.

To Alexander, your contribution and coaching acted as a bridge to finding my confidence and giving me a peek into who I am meant to be in this life. I love the life-changing wisdom you share that was hidden in the deck of playing cards. (www.lifeelevated.life)

To Rachel (www.racheltheastrologer.com), your priceless readings inspired the book title and so much more.

To my dear Ed, for finding me in this lifetime. How did I get so lucky? How does it get any better than this?

For you readers:

You will find questions as you peruse this book. The questions are asked not for an answer, but for awareness. In psychology, the term *awareness* is a concept of knowing, being, and perceiving something. It is tapping into your inner knowing, and being open to receiving that information.

Many of the questions in this book are inspired by Gary Douglas and Dr. Dain Heer, who are the founders of something called Access Consciousness® (www.accessconsciousness.com). Access Consciousness is a set of tools and processes that empower you to know what you know (that you didn't know you know).

I have found this modality to be tremendously easy to implement in my life and using it has created major shifts and lots of magic in so many ways. It's shown me how to clear the blocks that limit me, and then to tap into my own natural magic.

So many tools, and so much expanded awareness.

If I had to share a favorite, it might be the question "Who does this belong to?". Why that question? 98% of our thoughts, feelings, and emotions don't actually belong to us. What? Yep! They are just implanted points of view from the world around us that we have absorbed since infancy. Next time you get angry or judgmental ask yourself, "Who does this belong to?' You may be surprised that it's not even yours. Now you can say, send it back to the sender. It's just stuck energy. Keep doing that over and over and you will get lighter. Try it.

Another tool I love is "living" an "Interesting Point of View". What does that mean? It means no two people can share the exact same point of view because we all think a little differently, even when we think alike. This also means there is no right or wrong, it's just that we think differently and that's ok IF we allow it to be.

So when someone says something that triggers you, say silently or out loud, "Interesting point of view, you have that point of view".

One more great tool from Access Consciousness is "choosing greater" vs settling for what is.

I have learned that when you settle for less, you get less than you settled for.

How can we choose greater? Keep asking questions and keep choosing. There are no wrong choices. Just choices. Every choice creates something more.

All of these tools and my years of seeking happiness have made it so much easier to find the true purpose of my life which is to be happier and more creative and be a contribution to myself and the world.

This book is the first tangible gift I have created to share with others and is part of my personal exploration of Joy and Happiness.

So here are some questions for you to start your journey:

How can you use this book to your advantage?

What is possible beyond this reality that you've never considered before?

How much fun can you have today?

How did we get so lucky to be here together at this time?

Something wonderful is happening, how can we tap into it?

If today didn't have to be anything like the past, what could you choose and what could you create?

I wonder? Enjoy the journey!

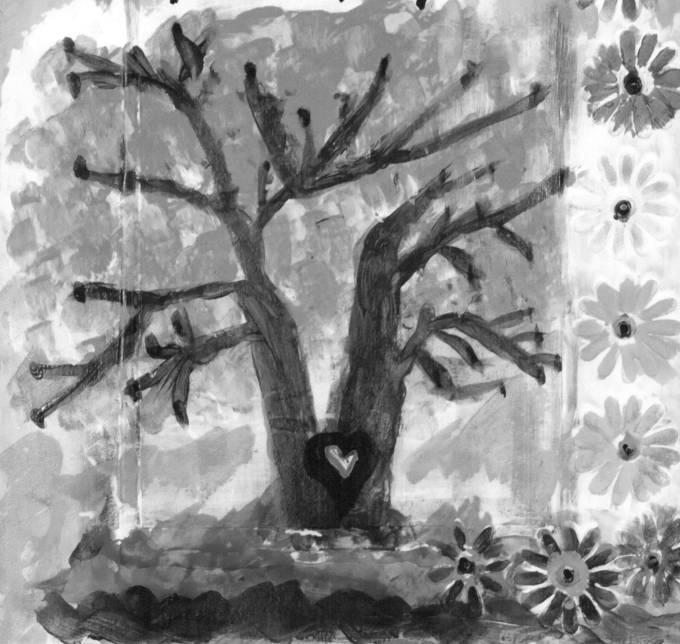

YOU ARE SO BEAUTIFUL

What if thinking well of yourself is the greatest act of kindness?

Paying attention to your thoughts will begin to eliminate those that don't serve you.

If your thoughts create your reality,
what will you tell yourself today?

LET IT GO

it's OK

YOU HAVE TO LOOK IN THE MIRROR and LIKE WHAT YOU SEE and THEN WHAT YOU SEE CAN CHANGE

STOP CRITICIZING YOUR-SELF

ACCEPT YOURSELF AS YOU ARE ♥

NOTES TO SELF

Note to Self:

Self-judgment is the biggest sin.
When we let go of that, we make space for
magic and miracles to come into our life.

What would it take for you to stay out of
self-judgment and move into self-love today?

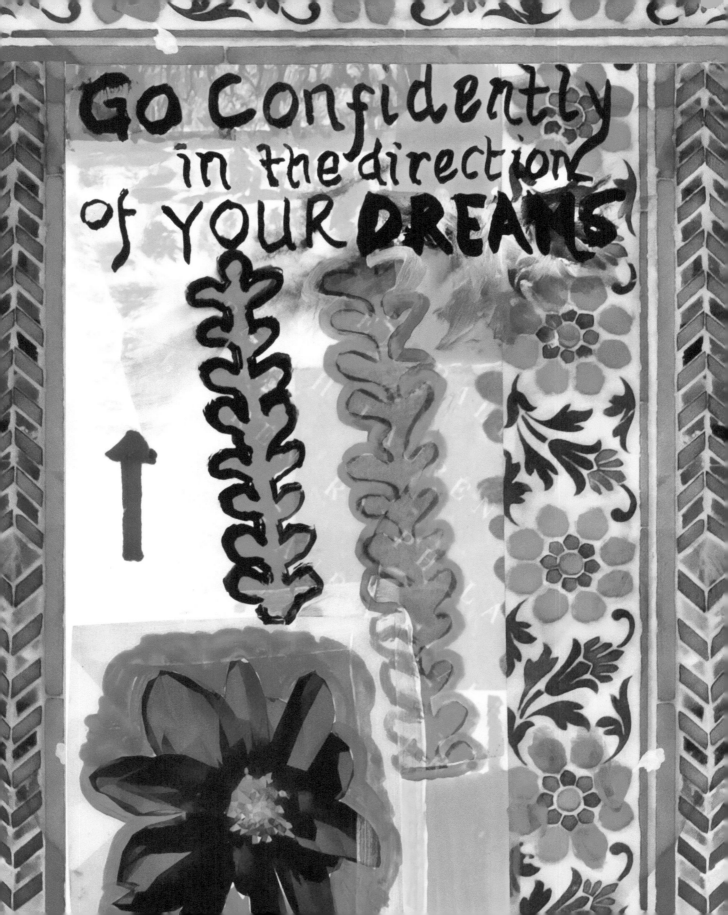

Which way do I go?

Go and be guided by the opportunities that show up all around you. Follow the ones that feel like a contribution to the life you are choosing to live.

Life is meant to be fun and adventurous.

What great and glorious adventures can you have today?

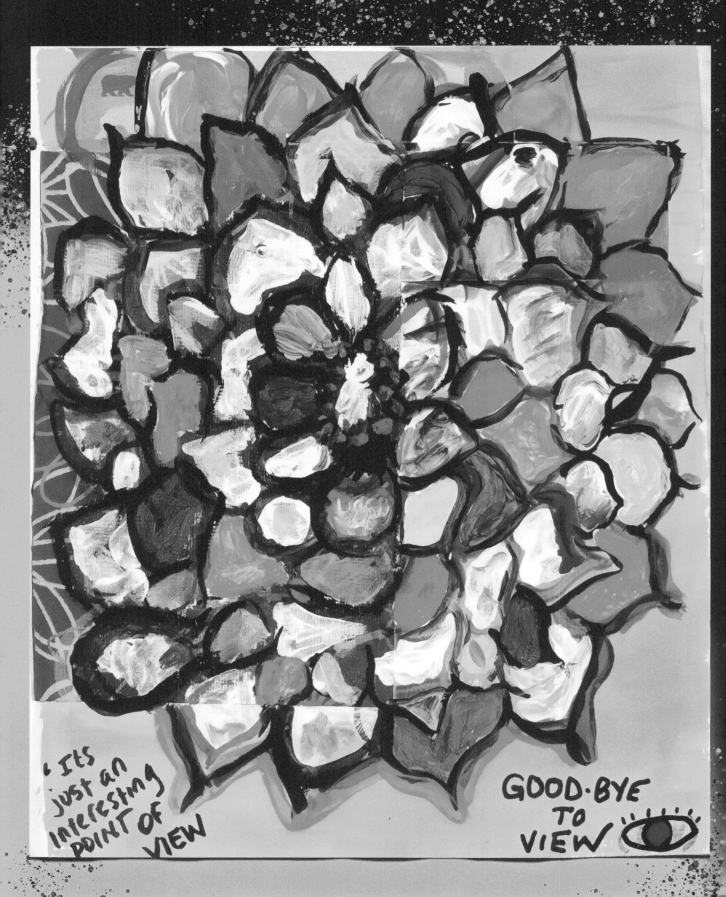

' Its just an interesting point of view

GOOD·BYE TO VIEW

Instead of being busy fighting for what's right or what's wrong, what if we started to see everything as an **interesting point of view?**

This is how we move into greater awareness. The greater the awareness we have, the greater access we have to energy and information.

Today, what if you see everything as just an interesting point of view?

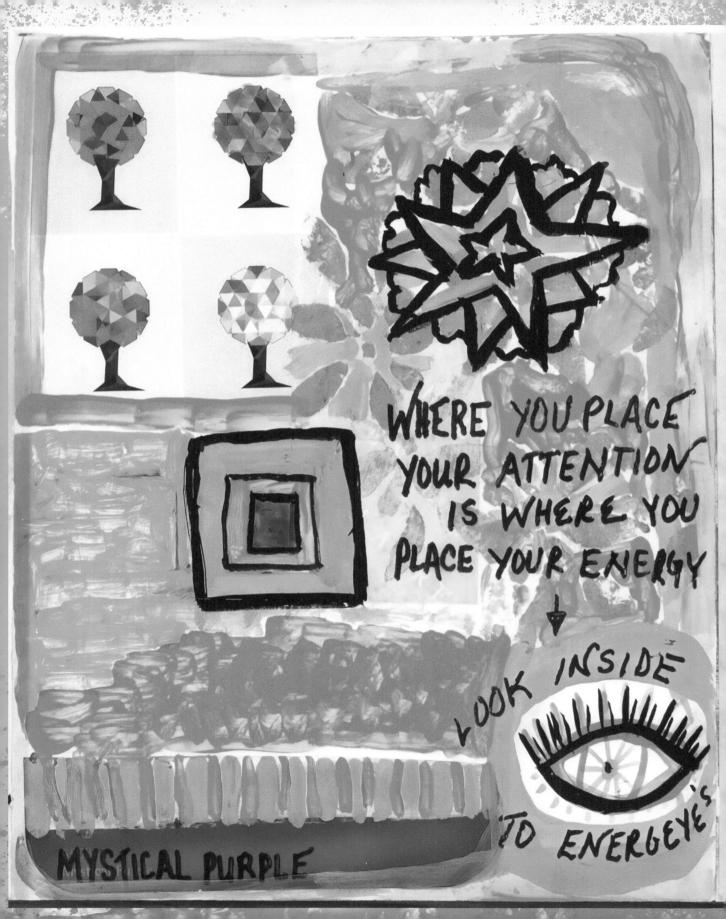

WHERE YOU PLACE
YOUR ATTENTION
IS WHERE YOU
PLACE YOUR ENERGY

LOOK INSIDE

TO ENERGEYE'S

MYSTICAL PURPLE

Energy flows where attention goes.

"When you change the way you look at things the things you look at change."
— Wayne Dyer

What can I see differently today for my world to show up in a brand new way?

ASK QUESTIONS:

that are open ended
where you are not looking
for a result.

What else is possible
that you have not yet
asked for?

what is valuable to you? what
do you actually give a shit about?

Are your choices supporting
"that" + creating "that" as a
possibility? ★ ★ ★ ★ ★

Chaos
Chaos
Order
Order

DON'T TRUST ME TRUST YOU

What if.. you were
meant to receive?

How many of you are not
willing to receive?

neither resist + react or align + agree
living in a world of no judgement
including you.

What if you saw a possibility
rather than a problem?

When I take time to nurture MYSELF. ☐
I SUPERCHARGE my own energy ☐

GOOD NEWS MATTERS

YOU Matter

How do you energetically feed yourself? Do you nurture yourself? Do you watch the news every day? Do you listen to people complain about the same things over and over?

The motivational speaker Jim Rohn famously said, "We are the average of the five people we spend the most time with".

Take inventory of who is around you.

Are they nurturing to you and feeding your well-being, or are they feeding your dis-ease?

I WISH I HAD DONE THAT

it's never too late!

ASK: WOULD THIS BE A CONTRIBUTION TO my LIFE?

IF YES, then ASK: what ACTION can I take to ACTUALIZE this?

Living Happily Ever After

I wish I had done that.

I wish I hadn't done that.

Either way, you can still choose something greater now.

Choice is your superpower.

What if it's never too late, you are never too old, you can't get it wrong and you will never get it done?

What can you choose now?

Meeting ID: 886 232 7777

Just for ME
just for FUN
I don't have to
TELL anyone

what does it take to make this a reality?

FOOD FOR THOUGHT

What other people think of you is none of your business.

What you think of you is your life's work. If you master this concept, you master your life.

Some people are just not ready for your choices, your awareness, and your greatness. That's OK. Don't let that stop you!

Today, what can you do that's just for you, just for fun and you don't have to tell anyone?

YOU WILL BE Among those who WILL SPREAD THE VIRUS OF WELL-BEING

awareness

optimism
Stability

The ELEGANCE of creation is using the least amount of effort to create the greatest Possibility

If you get happier,
the world gets happier.
Spread the virus of well-being.

Have fun.

Choose awareness.

Relax and receive.

How happy can you make you today?

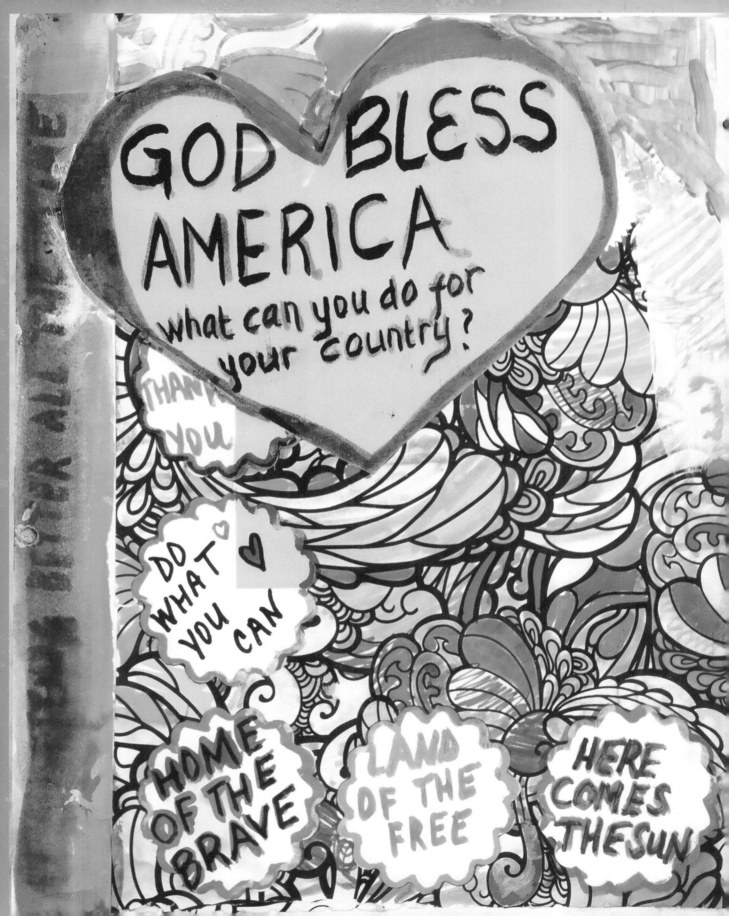

No matter where you are from or where you are living now, we all live in this world together. One world. One mother. Mother Earth. The most important state is our state of Being.

The more joyous that state is, the more joy we put into our world.

What if your JOY is what the world needs more of?

WHAT YOU BELIEVE IS WHAT YOU RECEIVE

WE ATTRACT HOW WE FEEL

I BELIEVE IN
Magic

I FEEL
Magical

STOP STOP
CANCEL
CLEAR
FEAR →EXIT→
GET OUT OF HERE

You don't have to believe in magic.

You are magic.

You have to believe in yourself, and then the magic happens.

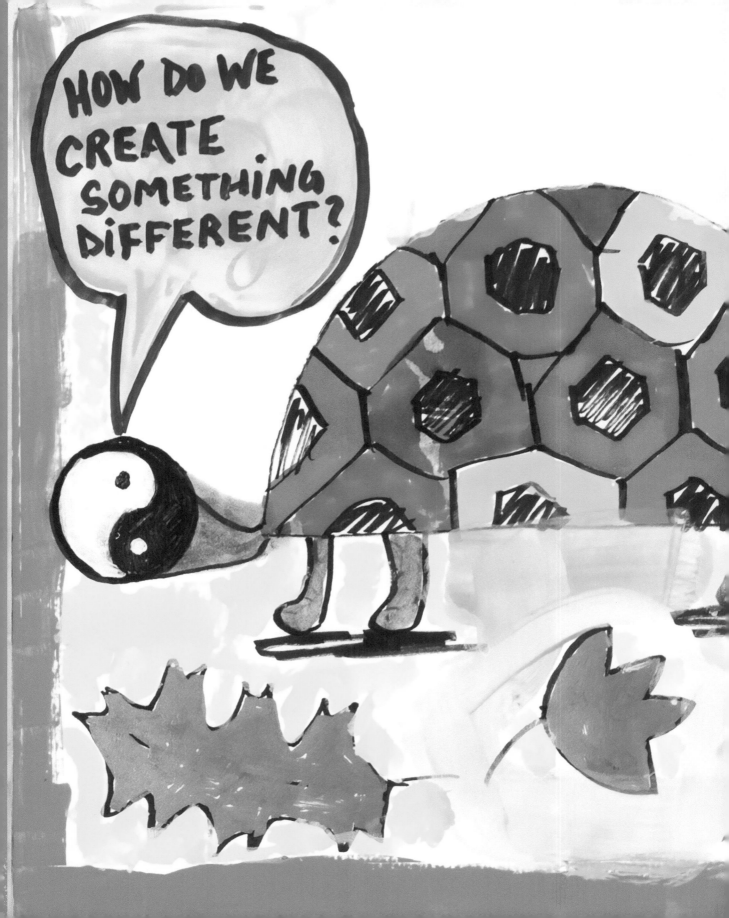

Rather than trying to prove what's right or wrong, there is another option: You can ask a question like:

How do we create something different?

When we take ourselves out of the judgment of right and wrong, we create space for new possibilities to show up.

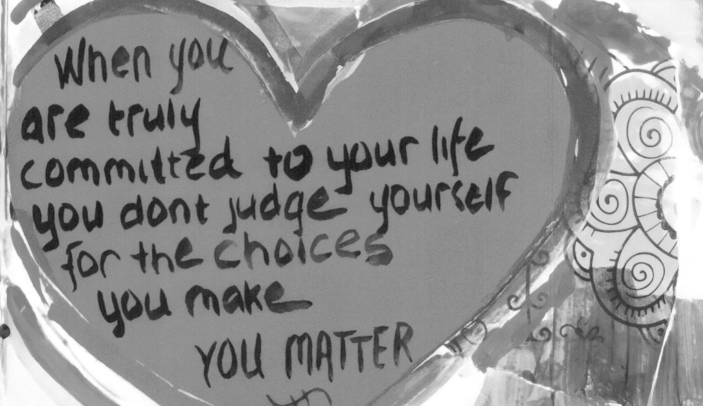

FREEDOM TO stand in your own truth regardless of what might HAPPEN

When you are truly committed to your life you dont judge yourself for the choices you make

YOU MATTER

True freedom is being free from the thoughts of judgment.

If you don't judge you, nobody else can either.

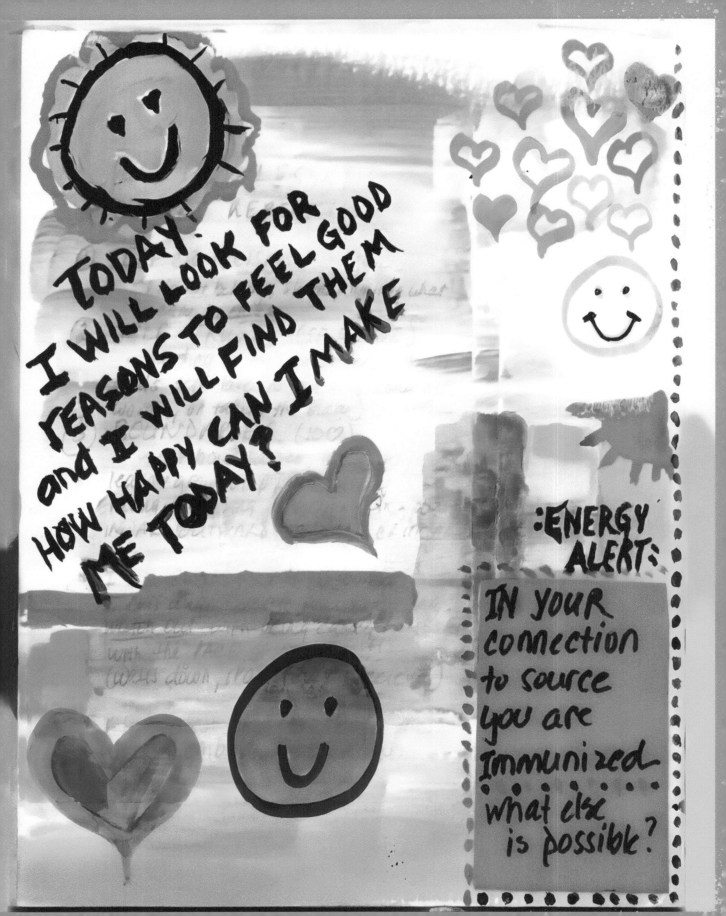

Happiness is a choice.

Misery is a choice.

It's just a choice.

You are the chooser!

What do you want to choose today?

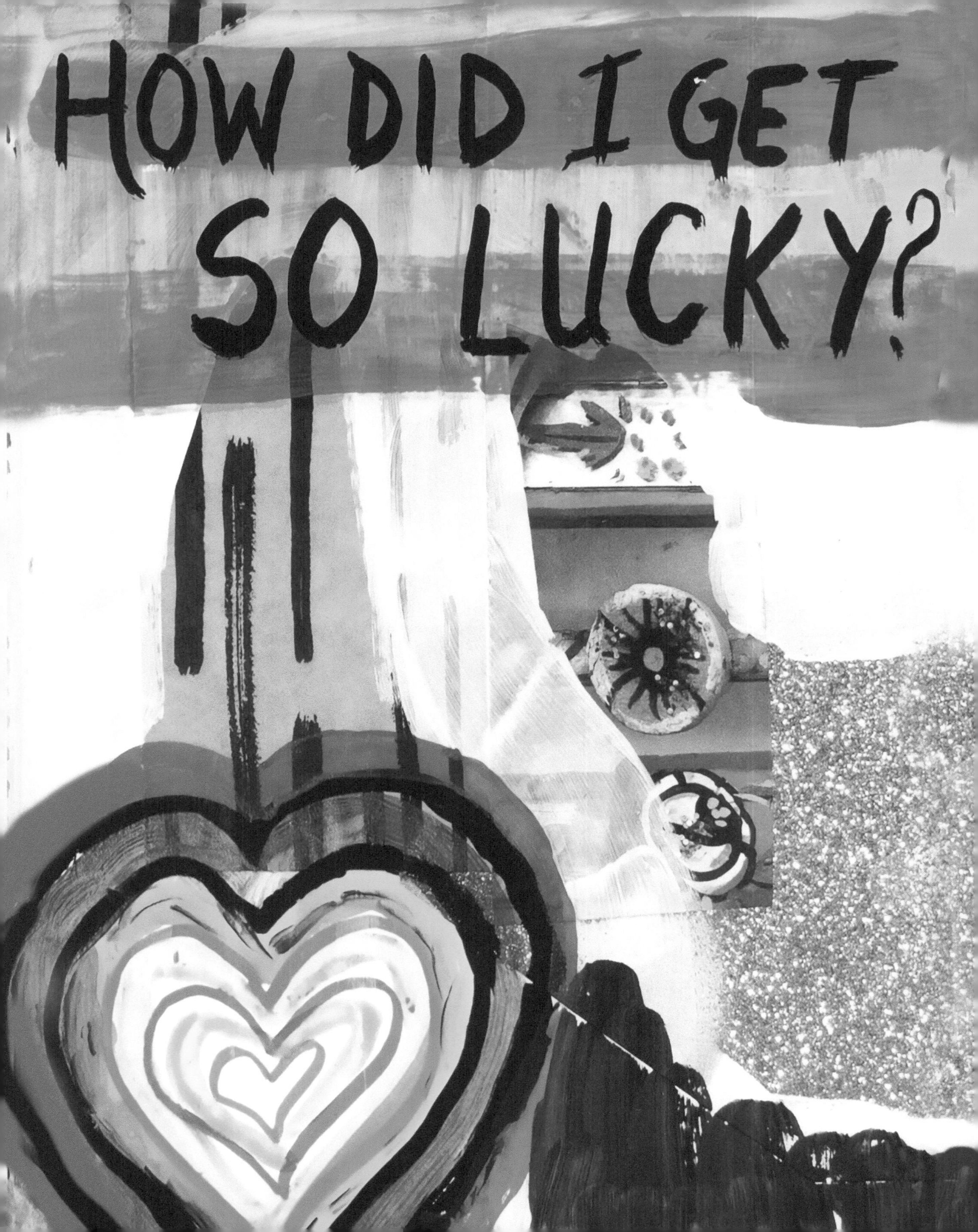
HOW DID I GET
SO LUCKY?

The attitude of gratitude

The more gratitude you have, the more you will have to be grateful for.

What you appreciate, appreciates.

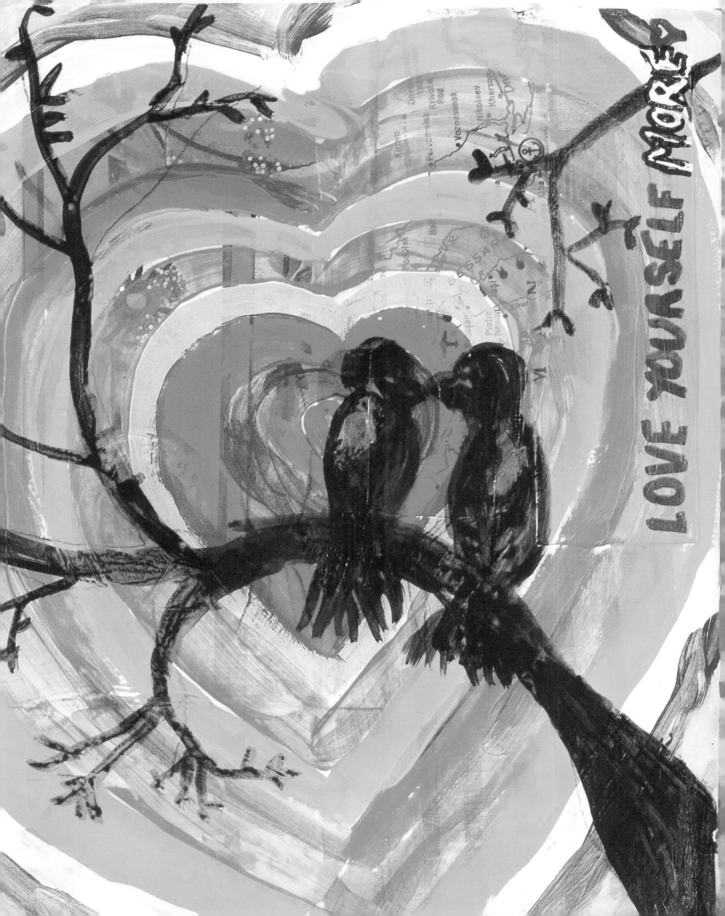

Love Yourself More

It's easy to get stuck in negative thought patterns. Those patterns create stress in our body and can cause dis-ease. On the flip side, research shows that people who think well of themselves have better physical and emotional health and are more resilient in times of stress. A positive mindset can lead to a thriving life. Affirmations are a great way to love yourself more.

I love myself, I am powerful, I am loved, I am beautiful, I am safe....

What kind words can you say to yourself today?

With my Luck
it will probably work
out and will-l
work out FASTER
- - - FOR ME - - -
It's GOOD - - -
and
It's TRUE ♡

What if, with your luck, everything is always working out for you?

What if something wonderful is always on the verge of happening?

What would it take for today to be one of the best days of your life?

The World has a way of defining you if you don't Know who you are when 'you' get out there

Hello World,

I am creating my life and I'll tell you who I am.

Who I am today is not the same as who I was yesterday.

We get to recreate ourselves every morning.

Who do you want to be today?

What choices can you make to create the you you want to be?

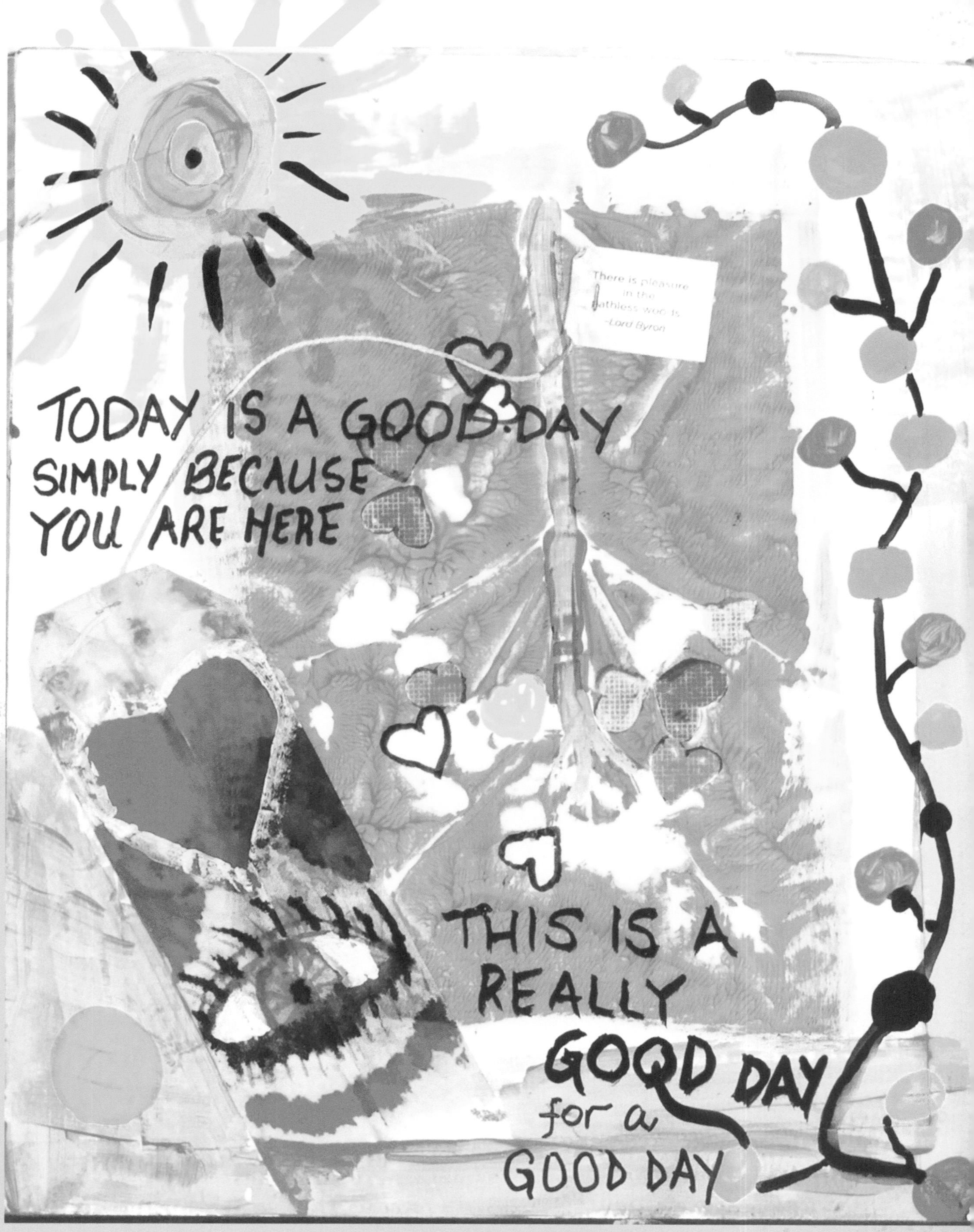
There is pleasure in the pathless woods
-Lord Byron
TODAY IS A GOOD DAY
SIMPLY BECAUSE
YOU ARE HERE
THIS IS A
REALLY
GOOD DAY
for a
GOOD DAY

What if the day you were born, the world knew it couldn't exist without you?

Today is a good day simply because you are here.

How can you celebrate you today?

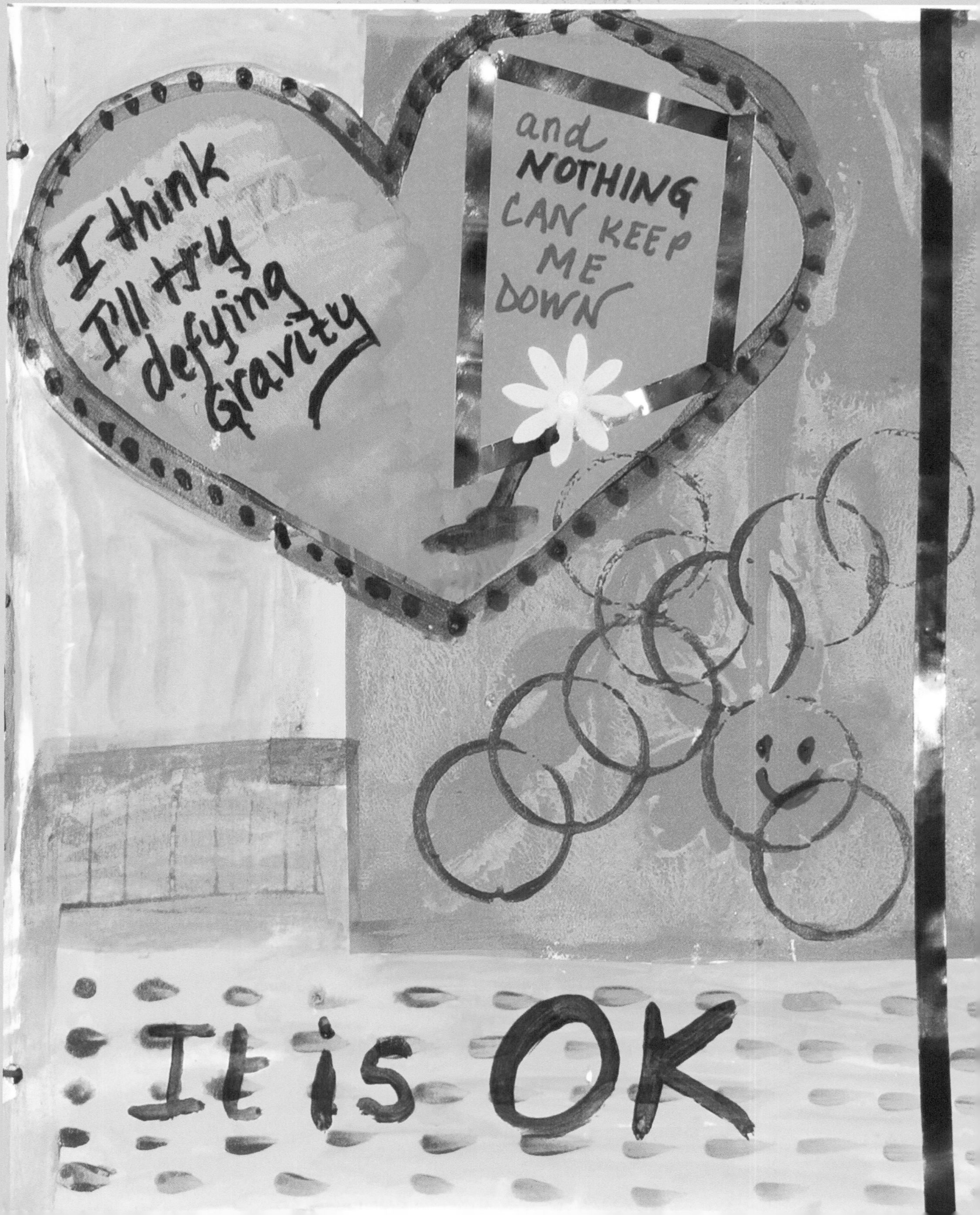
I think I'll try defying Gravity
and NOTHING CAN KEEP ME DOWN
It is OK

Don't let anyone dim your light,
not even you.

Turn it up.

You are here to shine!

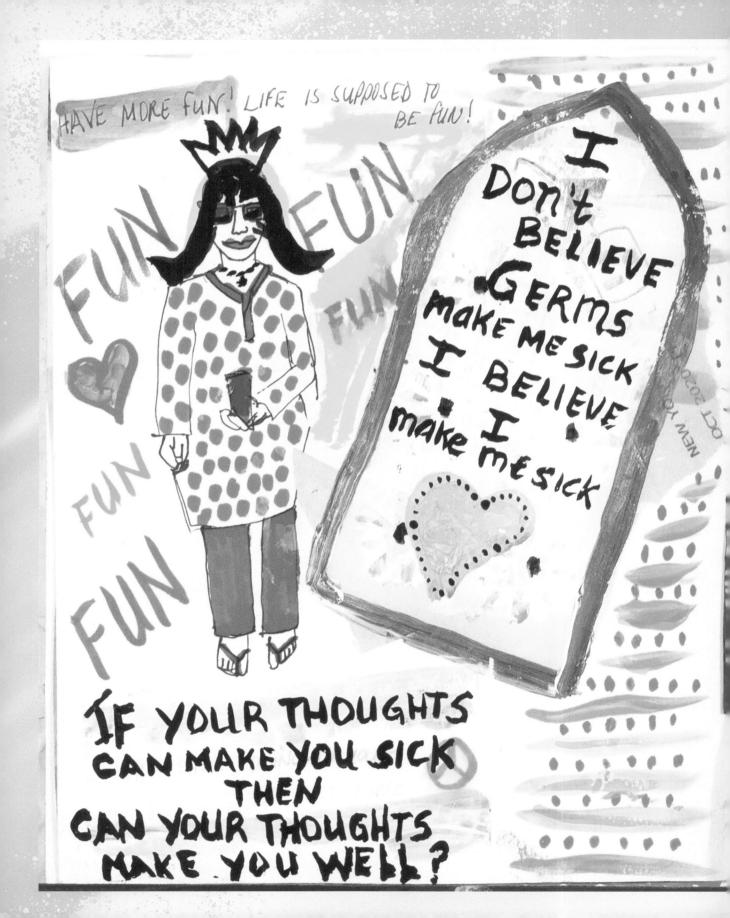

What if fun and joy is what keeps you well?

How does it get any better than that?

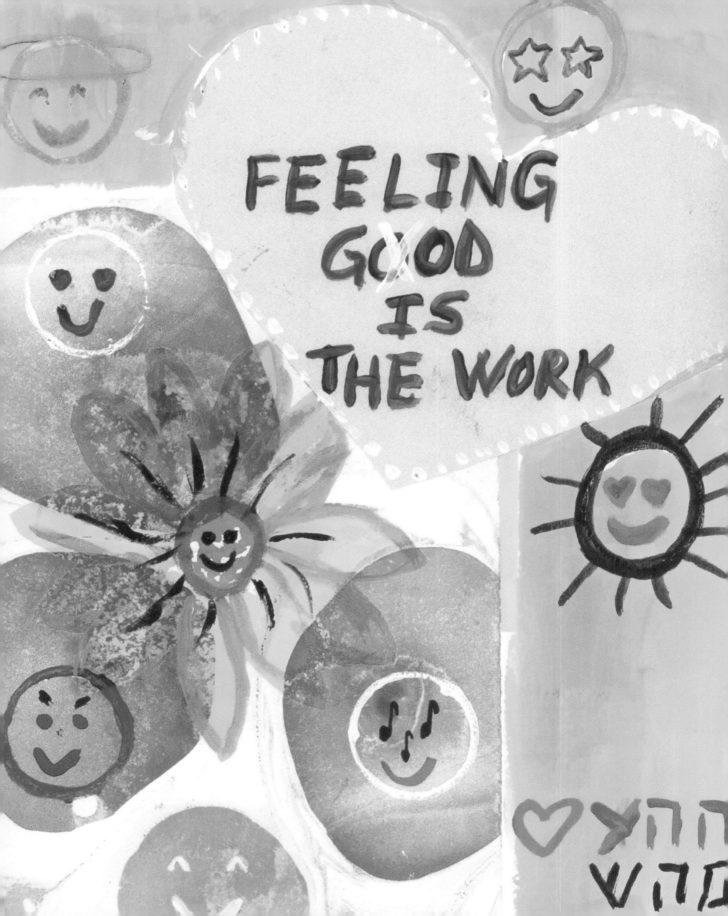

Good, Energy, God, Space, Magic, Higher Power, Miracle, Mystical, Inner Being, Universe, Creator, Infinite Being.

Call it what you wish.

You are all of it.

Be it.

Create with it.

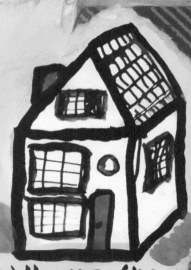

www.theverafter.com

Sometimes the
BEST SECRETS
are kept by
sharing them with
the world :)

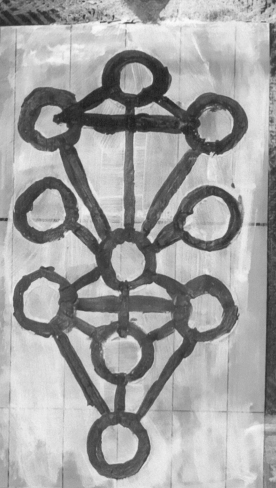

Keeping a secret is a way of separating you from others. That is why many ancient wisdoms were kept secret. To keep them separate and protected. The world wasn't ready, and people who held the secrets were at risk of being killed.

Well, those days are over!

There is magical wisdom everywhere. All you have to do is ask, be curious and it will show up, then receive it.

You did that with this book.

What secrets do you know?

Be there for yourself
don't scare yourself with
FRIGHTFUL THOUGHTS

You are the CREATOR
of your own reality

POWER

You are a powerful creator.
Choosing is your creative superpower.

If you know every choice creates something, what will you choose today?

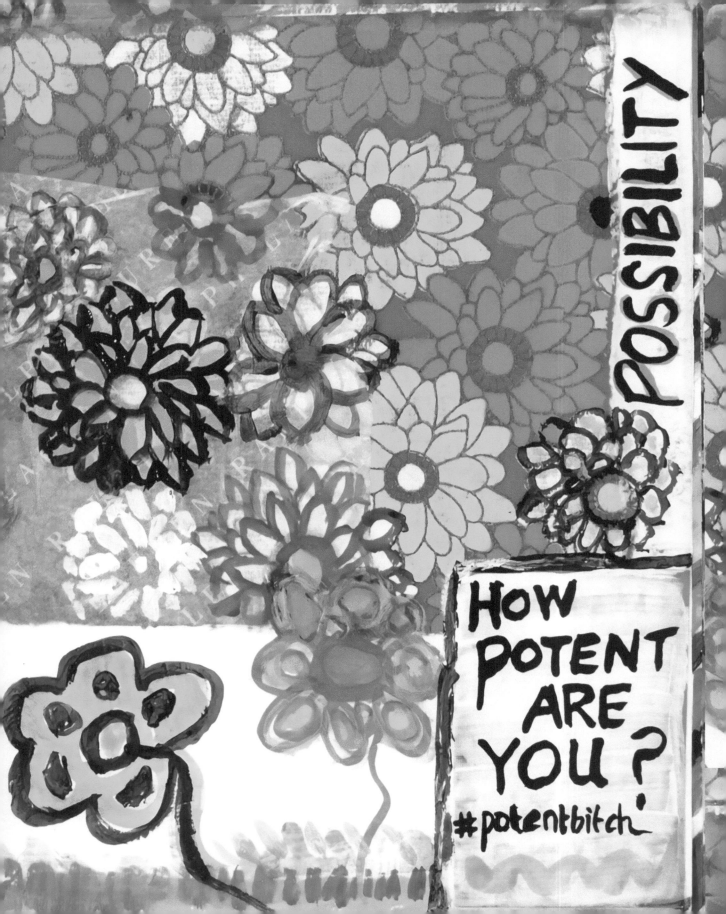

POSSIBILITY

HOW
POTENT
ARE
YOU?
#potentbitch

People often say,
"Who am I to do that? Why me?"

Actually,

why not you?

About the Author

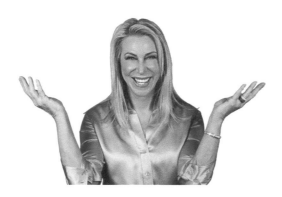

Donna Jane Sirlin is an author and happiness seeker who helps anyone ready to shift their mindset. A certified Access Bars practitioner, Reiki Healer, and Breath Coach. Donna is a grateful wife to Ed and her children, who bring so much joy to her world.

To learn more about Donna and her work, email Donna.Sirlin@gmail.com or follow her on Instagram @healing.through.happiness.

Notes: